The Menopause Mindshift

The Menopause Mindshift

How I Unleashed My Inner Queen, And You Can Too!

Lisa R. Triggs

This book was printed in the United States of America.
Order additional copies of this book from Amazon.com.

www.themenopausemindshift.com

ISBN (paperback): 978-1-0690254-1-8
ISBN (ebook): 978-1-0690254-0-1

Book design and production by www.AuthorSuccess.com
Cover art by www.stock.adobe.com

Disclaimer
This book is a personal account of my experiences and reflections. The narratives and stories shared within are based solely on my individual journey and are not intended to provide medical advice or represent universal experiences of menopause or any other life events discussed. I am not a medical professional or expert in the fields of health, psychology, or related disciplines. Readers are encouraged to consult qualified health care professionals for advice and information regarding their specific circumstances. The views and opinions expressed in this book are my own and do not claim to reflect the experiences or views of others undergoing similar life stages or situations.

*For women everywhere
who are ready to shift how
they think about menopause*

My body is in
perfect balance
at all times

Contents

*I embrace
my evolving self
with love and
compassion*

Introduction

*I*f I were a time traveller and could go back in time, I would tell myself this: 'Don't let menopause symptoms make you stray from being the best you can be! Stay focused on you because you are the key to everything.'

Having gone through it, I would give the same advice now to any woman about to enter her menopause years.

There came a period where I found myself giving other women pep talks about their menopause symptoms, even when I was having a difficult time myself. I hid what was truly going on inside of myself from the outside world the best I could. I encouraged women to find something good about menopause and focus on that. Not having to cart around pads or tampons is a good thing, right?

As I was going through my metamorphosis, it became clear that I should share my story and the transformation I underwent. No woman should have to struggle as I did! No woman should struggle as I allowed myself to!

I discovered that by putting into practice, the things I was already familiar with, I was able to improve my menopause symptoms. I realized that the more I explored the various mediums available, the more I shed what did not serve me, allowing me to improve my menopause symptoms and feel alive again. My only wish is that I had been in a place to connect the dots years earlier because I could have avoided so much misery.

This book is a narrative of my journey and the tools I used to improve my menopause symptoms by using my thoughts and mindset. I battled feelings of fatigue, depression, anger, sleeplessness and a laundry list of other symptoms for almost seven years before I recognized that I had possessed the power to change things in myself the whole time!

Like so many other women, I have considered my menopause years to be nothing short of awful. It has been a road I wouldn't wish on anyone. I was having a difficult time in my relationships with my spouse, God, the universe, and making sense of my entire life. I experienced a list of almost thirty symptoms, some of which I would have never thought had anything to do with menopause. It has been a very strange time, which included an unexpected twist involving my husband.

Let me ask you this: How many other women can say that their husbands had their own hormone issues during menopause?

Not long after I began full menopause, my husband was diagnosed with a pituitary tumour. The pituitary gland plays a crucial role in regulating various physiological processes by secreting hormones that control other glands in the endocrine system. In English, it produces several essential hormones that help regulate the body. In women, it helps to regulate our milk production and aids in controlling our reproductive system, among other things. In men, it produces growth hormone, stimulates the production of testosterone, and regulates water balance, for example.

When the pituitary gland isn't functioning properly in a man, many complications can occur, one of which is the increased production of prolactin. If the prolactin level is too high in a man, it leads to a host of issues, including erectile dysfunction, decreased libido, infertility, and sometimes gynecomastia (enlargement of breast tissue in men).

I would have never fathomed that the diagnosis of his tumour would end up affecting my life as much, or more as it did my husbands. He was put on medication that is typically used to treat Parkinson's disease, but as a side effect, also reduces pituitary tumours. The medication affected his behaviour, and as a result, I fell into a deep depression. This went on for five years before we learned that there were side effects we weren't aware of, and he stopped taking it. The new side effects we learned about included gambling addiction, sex addiction, impulse control issues, and ADHD-like behaviours. Funny thing is, when you look up the drug online, you don't see anything about those effects.

The fun didn't stop there, though!

After discontinuing the medication, he exhibited symptoms of being in menopause as well, or andropause. That's the male version of menopause. His hormones and moods fluctuated like a yoyo, going up and down, up and down, sometimes spinning out of control. He wasn't alone though; I was going through the same thing. That was my life.

Some days, he was overly sensitive. Others he wanted to take on the world. What could we do? What else was there to help reduce or destroy this tumour? There were some days his symptoms were worse than mine and it was almost unbearable. We were both walking on eggshells, trying our best to maintain some sort of normal life even though it was in chaos.

After a lot of discussion on how to proceed, we settled on testosterone gel, which took some time to adjust the dosage. In the meantime, though, our lives were a constant hormonal roller coaster that didn't ever stop to let us; or me, off. There were sugar cravings, lethargy, ADHD symptoms, trouble sleeping, feeling tired, weight gain, negativity, and countless other things going on. And that was just my husband!

My life felt so stressful. For years, my life has revolved around my husband. He was diagnosed with celiac disease in 2011, which means we must always choose places he can go to. He hates it, because where we eat, where we travel, whose house we go to, it's always about him!

Can't he get something that can be cured? I know it's not easy on him, but I just wanted some peace in my life without having to worry about someone else's issues for a while. Calgon, take me away!

All women go through this phase of life. For some, it's a breeze; for others, it's more difficult. In my opinion, mine has been a nightmare. It felt like I was on the run from my life. I was lethargic and tired, just going through the motions of everyday life. I was stressed out by my husband's condition and gained almost forty pounds. I had trouble sleeping at night and had no desire for intimacy, which put a strain on my marriage.

As time went on, new symptoms arose, which left me feeling like I was literally living in hell. Things that I had no idea could be related to menopause started happening, like feelings of electric shock and rage.

I was surprised to find what an extensive list of menopause symptoms there was! I was even more stunned to read how many on the list I had. Out of thirty-one initial menopause symptoms on the list I found, I had all but one. That was in 2022, and since then, I have come across other lists that have forty and up to one hundred symptoms. Yikes! I was doomed!

After over seven years of feeling miserable, I wanted off the roller coaster I was on. Life was passing me by. I started searching for new versions of old habits. I have been big on the law of attraction and practicing gratitude for years. I bought any new book put out by Rhonda Byrne, author of *The Secret*, that I could find and started absorbing every positive vibe I could, but with new eyes.

It had been years since I picked up the original *Secret* book, and I wanted to expand my horizons. I was interested to see what new things Rhonda had to say, and I found exactly what I was looking for. Little did I know that this would just be the beginning of a complete transformation. It wasn't just books that turned me on, though. I started to piece together things I had been missing in my previous practices, so I started implementing affirmations, music, and meditation into my daily life.

One day, I remembered that there were different frequencies of music that were supposed to help with specific areas, like stress, love, anxiety, and money. The music can be found on YouTube, so I started searching for any, and all frequencies that pertained to my life. That was the beginning of the new me! I put the old and new routines together for a combination that changed everything for me.

While at a therapy session, the topic of guided meditation came up, so I searched YouTube and found a twenty-minute guided meditation by Bob Proctor, renowned self-help author, motivational speaker, and success coach of the Proctor-Gallagher Institute. The meditation focuses on creating abundance in your life using the law of vibration. I loved it! I did as Bob instructed in the meditation and listened every day for at least thirty days.

I learned more about the law of vibration. I was only familiar with the law of attraction, but the law of vibration is actually the second law, while the law of attraction is the fourth. During meditation, you can become in tune with the law of vibration, and when you do that, you are in a place where you can envision how you want your life to be.

I incorporated the meditation into my daily gratitude, and I started to feel different. I incorporated listening to the frequency music while I wrote my gratitude list and journal entry for the day. It included how I was feeling, what goals I might have for the day, or anything I needed to get off my chest. It was one of the best things I did for myself and do for myself still.

Every woman should know how to do this. No woman should struggle, not being who she truly is and living the fullest life she can, not just during her menopause years, but at any time. It is one of the easiest ways I found to improve my symptoms, and even eradicate some altogether. After years of counselling and therapy on my own and with my husband, I did more in a few months of focusing on the right things, than I had in years of therapy.

I am sharing my personal transformative journey with the hope that other women might find a path forward, as well. I hope each reader takes away something new they hadn't thought of before. My hope is that my story helps you improve yours.

By no means am I suggesting that anyone go off their medication, stop therapy or other treatment they may be currently undertaking. Don't stop any exercise routine or healthy eating plan that you are on. I believe that all these things are very helpful. Instead, I advocate adding these practices into your daily routine to see where it takes you.

This book is about finding yourself and unleashing the person you were always meant to be. It's about shifting the way you think and choosing to be in control of your life. Each chapter is meant to take you on my journey of self-discovery as well as your own.

I have had experience with many mediums, each having their own value and impact on the journey from where I was to where I am now.

My hope is that after reading this book, you learn how to permanently shift your menopause mindset, or as I call it, undergo a menopause mindshift.

I want you to know that if I can do this, you can too! You are not alone. You have more power over your thoughts than you think, and you are stronger than you think you are.

I want every woman to know that we don't just have to survive this time in our lives, we can thrive, too! My mission is to empower every woman to think of herself as a Queen during menopause. That thought alone raises the vibration and sets you on a positive path.

I want you to know that there will be setbacks and that it can take time. It's okay if you have a bad day, just start fresh again the next. I want you to be patient WITH yourself and kind TO yourself and as others.

Most of all, I hope you feel love. Love is the key to so much of our lives, even when we can't see it.

During this past year, I discovered the value of loving myself and remembering the things I loved about the people in my life. I was stuck in a negative narrative that I thought was my life, and it took me far too long to snap out of it.

I now live by the mantra: *I must change things IN me to change things FOR me.*

It all begins and ends with me. It always has and always will. It all begins and ends with you, too, and it always will.

You always have a choice each day when you wake up and get out of bed. You always choose how your day goes, good or bad. You set the tone for your day and your life. It's your choice, and that's the beauty of it!

Choose to love, even when it's hard. Choose to speak to others with respect, even when they have wronged you. Choose to sing and be happy, even when you feel low. Choose to forgive, even when you don't want to.

Remember, 'your thoughts become things.'

If your thoughts become things, then when you think good thoughts, good things happen, and it can be as simple as that. It is true: you are the master of your own destiny.

Drink the Kool-Aid! Drink up as much as you can and share it with everyone. Buy in. Invest in yourself because you are worth it.

Affirm yourself and trust who you are. Know that all good is coming to you and that you are attracting all good into your life.

Tell yourself you are a lucky girl and that you deserve all you desire.

Remember that you are strong, powerful, and you are enough! Remind yourself that menopause is just a phase of life; it's not your life, and it's not forever.

Believe that your menopause journey is easy. Tell your hormones to be in perfect balance.

You can do it! You can use your mindset to improve your symptoms and your life to be the Queen you were meant to be. Don't hide her. Let her out for all to see. Don't just survive menopause. Thrive during it!

*Menopause
is a time of renewal
and new beginnings
for me*

CHAPTER ONE

A Transformative Year

Calling all the beautiful menopausal Queens who are walking the Earth! Your inner Queen is in there, so let her loose!

Would you believe me if I told you, that you could improve your menopause symptoms by simply shifting your mindset? It worked for me, and I believe it can work for you, as well.

I am calling 2023 my transformative year. I discovered myself in a whole new way that has been liberating and feels so inherently good. It wasn't all roses. In fact, it was an emotional rollercoaster. But what I uncovered about myself and what I could do with my own thoughts has been so empowering that it's hard to contain it!

When I look back at who I was before 2023, I was lost for over seven years. I didn't recognize the person looking back at me in the mirror any longer. Who was this woman?

This woman had a double chin, and her face was round, but mine had always been thin. Her eyes looked sullen and lacked lustre, and she had bags underneath them with dark circles.

The woman in the mirror had a belly that looked as if she was five months pregnant, but I was always thin and trim, even after having two children.

This woman lost her balance and was out of breath climbing a flight of stairs. She was fearful and sad. She gained almost forty pounds and believed that no matter what she did, she; could not lose it.

This woman just wanted to be alone. She couldn't handle crowds anymore and everything overwhelmed her. Even the simplest of tasks seemed way too much.

She cried at the drop of a hat. There was a period where she cried daily for three months straight. She had immense anger about everything and no patience whatsoever. This woman lacked zest for life and was just going through the motions of everyday life. She was faking it!

She had no desire for intimacy and didn't care about taking care of anyone but herself. She was experiencing frequent urinary and yeast infections, and everything was dry, if you know what I mean.

She would pee her pants when she sneezed and for some reason her teeth ached.

She was moody and irritable, swinging from 'I love you' to 'Don't come near me' and 'Maybe we should separate,' then back to 'I don't want to separate,' all in one day.

The woman I saw looking back at me was looking tired and hadn't had a good night's sleep in so long that she couldn't remember when.

Hot flashes were a nightly occurrence, sometimes drenching her nightclothes and bed. All she wanted to do was nothing. She was tired all the time.

The woman I was looking at in the mirror could not focus on any one task at a time. Her mind would race from thought to thought like a bee fluttering from flower to flower and she couldn't remember what she was doing in the first place.

She would forget things she just said and couldn't remember what she did yesterday, let alone the week earlier.

Feeling stressed was a daily occurrence for this woman. Her hair was thinning and falling out. Her fingernails became brittle. She experienced ongoing vertigo and dizziness for months on end.

This woman was suddenly pre-diabetic. How? She had been

hypoglycemic for years, but now her blood sugar was unstable, and she craved carbs and sugar all the time.

Who was this woman I saw in the mirror? She just felt like a freight train had run over her again and again with no indication of when it would pull into the station.

This woman experienced tingling feelings like static shock throughout her body on a daily basis.

There were times when she thought she was crazy. She started to think about an exit plan, to put herself and everyone else out of misery.

Then, studying the woman in the mirror more closely, it suddenly hit me. The woman in the mirror was me!

Was I having an out-of-body experience? Nope. This was my life during menopause. To say it has been unique is an understatement. Some days, it felt like I was living someone else's life in someone else's body, not my own.

I was thirty-eight when I started perimenopause. I knew something was going on when I started gaining a few pounds and couldn't get it off. My upper body was thickening, and my bra size began to increase. I tried to combat it by working out and watching what I ate, and for a little while I seemed to hold steady. I was in perimenopause for approximately ten years.

I was forty-seven when I hit full menopause and started to see a few more symptoms creep up. My cycles stopped, which I didn't mind, and I seemed to be going through a hormone burst, which my husband didn't mind.

Then, I began having mild hot flashes, so I bought some herbal supplements that did the trick.

I thought, Great! This isn't so bad. It's manageable.

The following year, I put on a few more pounds. Then again, the next. It was gradual until I turned fifty. By my fiftieth birthday in 2018, I had gained almost forty pounds, and my belly was extended and bloated as if I were pregnant. Which I was not! It was quite the opposite.

Life had changed drastically. It became complicated and stressful, and the herbal supplements just weren't cutting it anymore. I was having hot flashes multiple times every night. The insomnia started, so I was up until about 3:00 a.m. most nights. Of course, I also had to get up to pee at least once during the night, as well.

The one thing I was in no way prepared for was the mental health issues I have had, or that my spouse's hormones would have an impact on my experience in the way it did. It is unquestionably a unique situation when your spouse and you are going through menopause at the same time.

The diagnosis of the pituitary tumour changed everything. The side effects of the medication made him a different person, and life felt miserable to me most days.

Anxiety and depression became a significant part of my life, and there were many days when I felt overwhelmed. I thought I was going crazy, literally! It was as if I drove to crazy town, went around and around searching for the exit to leave, but couldn't find it. My life was out of control. It took me far too long to realize that it didn't have to be that way.

I learned valuable lessons the hard way to find the right path for me. Knowing that hormone therapy wasn't for me, especially after two years of trying it, was a significant step. When my doctor explained that prolonged use would make it harder to stop, I decided it wasn't the best choice for me. I preferred my body to rely on its natural hormone production rather than medication.

I was somewhat naive about menopause, not realizing the extensive range of symptoms. Like many women, I was unprepared, expecting just a few hot flashes. The reality was much more challenging, and no one had prepared me for it. The lack of preparation added to the difficulty, and I didn't truly understand what it would be like until I experienced it.

Various stressors in my life contributed to a challenging period. These external factors exacerbated my feelings, and I allowed them to affect me deeply. I reached a point where my motivation waned, and my primary goal became just getting through the workday to relax. During this time, doing very little felt comfortable, but it left me feeling disconnected and lost.

Everything in my life blended to create a recipe for disaster. All the outside stressors made everything worse, and I allowed them to. I was in a place where I had little desire to do much. I just wanted to get through my workday so I could relax on the couch and watch TV. Doing a lot of nothing was just fine with me! I felt completely lost.

In April 2011, I turned forty-four and had been in perimenopause for almost six years. In addition to what I was already dealing with, April also brought circumstances that would change our lives forever.

My father was seventy-six and in good health, overall. He had a bout with colon cancer a couple of years earlier but seemed to be in a good place health-wise at the time. He was strong and active, and a good man, but he had also always been a worrier. He was also the father of seven children, of which I am the youngest. Five of the seven are girls, so it's not surprising that he worried.

He started having headaches and getting dizzy, and after this went on for a few weeks, my mother finally convinced him to go to the doctor. They did some tests, and the diagnosis was brain cancer. He had two high-grade tumours in his head, and it was devastating news. Who survives brain cancer?

It's funny how you think about your parents living forever. He came through the colon cancer okay, so there was no reason to believe that he wouldn't beat this too, right? It really didn't sink in until he went in for a biopsy. Doctors wanted to see what the situation was exactly, so in they went. Dad was going to fight it, though. He started doing testing to see if he could withstand chemo to shrink these fuckers. But then he started to feel unwell, and his head was hurting. This went on for a few weeks until he finally collapsed and was taken to the hospital. After taking him in for surgery again, it was determined that they had nicked something when they performed the biopsy, and it had hemorrhaged. What the . . .?!?!

After the surgery, he lay in the hospital bed, and we were all unsure of what to do next. He was coherent and still of sound mind but was put on a lot of medication for the pain in his head. The pain was almost constant now, and no one knew what was going to happen to him. We didn't know how long he would be incapacitated or if he would need care, so he took that burden away from us. He said he wanted to be unhooked from the IV. He didn't want to put my mother or us kids through having to see him in this vegetative state. He died on the afternoon of June 18, 2011, at approximately 2:15 p.m. I spent his last two nights with him, and I feel so honoured to have done so.

My dad was cremated, and his urn laid to rest in a plot he and my mother had purchased for the two of them to spend eternity together.

You never really know how much you will miss a parent until they are gone. His death hit me harder than I ever expected it would. It all happened so fast. It was a two-month period from diagnosis to his passing. I felt this hole in my heart and still do, to this day.

That wasn't all that was going on, unfortunately. While we were going through this with my father, in April, my mother-in-law was admitted to the hospital, and they didn't really know what was wrong. My husband had always been close with his mum, so it was hard on him not to know what was wrong. At first, they thought her kidneys were failing, but then determined it was her heart. She was put on a list to see a heart specialist but remained in the hospital because she had become very weak.

We lived about three hours away in 2011, so we were back and forth quite a bit between our two parents. Then, at about 9:00 p.m. on May 31, the phone rang, and it was the hospital calling. Mum was suddenly declining, so they suggested that we come as soon as we could. We packed up the kids, who were seventeen and fourteen at the time, and hit the road.

We arrived just after midnight and all spent time with her. The hospital provided respite rooms, so we let the kids get some sleep while my husband and I sat with Mum. We really didn't know what was happening. It still wasn't that clear what the issue was or why she had taken such a turn for the worst.

We sat by her side, and around 3:00 a.m., we both were starting to fall asleep when I heard a big exhale. I popped up and nudged my husband. What was that? It had been her last breath. Mum passed on June 1, 2011. Oh, and she was still on the list for the heart specialist. They called a few months later with an appointment. Wow!

We each lost a parent within two weeks of each other. Both had gone from diagnosis to death in the same two-month stretch, April to June. We went through the motions of wakes and funerals. My husband was his mother's executor, so he had to take care of making her arrangements, which was hard on him. It was a lot to deal with for all of us.

It was such a painful time. I do not think either of us has ever really recovered from it. You try your best to be there for each other, but somehow what you need gets lost, so you just move forward. You push the pain down, put your big pants on, and get on with it, as the British say, all the while leaving a trail of emotional baggage that goes on for miles.

There was a long time afterward, when I felt like there was some resentment towards me, and I used to feel guilty. Then I realized that I was going through my own tough time, and I needed caring for, as well. I couldn't be the only one who was there for someone else as they grieved. I was grieving, too.

For years, I was convinced it was outside circumstances that caused me to feel the way I did. It couldn't all be just menopause, could it?

The more I've learned about menopausal symptoms in the last few years, the more I wonder if everything has just been a total mindfuck! Has menopause messed me up that much, or was I messed up to begin with? The jury's still out!

While going through it, I was sure that what was happening in my personal life amplified the symptoms. It made sense. I was under constant stress, I had become fearful, I had lost two parents, and I was living with a person I did not recognize anymore.

It has been a bumpy road back to wellness, and my inner voice still wonders what I ever did wrong to deserve this hell I have been through. However, I am so glad that I made it to the other side! Once I got here, life has been so much different.

I consider the path I chose to be a transformative journey because I have uncovered so much strength and resilience within myself. My life was upside down, and I was dangling by a thread before I recognized and embraced the power, I had all along. This journey has been a profound revelation, showing me that even in my darkest moments, I possessed an inner fortitude I never knew existed. Each challenge I faced became a stepping stone, leading me to a deeper understanding of my capabilities and potential.

Through this process, I discovered the importance of self-compassion and patience. I learned to navigate through the turbulence with a renewed sense of hope and determination. The trials and tribulations

I endured were not in vain; they were essential in shaping the person I am today.

I want to shout from the rooftops, 'Women of the world, if I can do this, so can you!' My journey has instilled in me a passion to inspire and empower others. I passionately believe that every woman has the strength within her to overcome adversity and emerge stronger. I hope to encourage others to embark on their own transformative journeys. I pray that they too uncover their hidden strengths, let go of any misconceptions they might have about menopause and create the most beautiful years of their lives yet.

*I honour the changes
in my body
during menopause*

CHAPTER TWO

Mind Control and Meditation

Something was missing, but I couldn't quite put my finger on it at first. I had to begin somewhere, so I decided to go back to my roots. Though I was still writing a gratitude journal each morning, it wasn't enough. I was ready to do more.

Meditation was the first form of manifestation I was introduced to, and it continues to be a driving force in my daily conscious awareness. Meditation was the anchor I was looking for to get my life on track.

I was introduced to mind control, which could be labeled as a form of meditation, around 1997. In the mid nineties, 1995, I think it was, we moved away from a small town to the big city. I was in the Big Smoke now, so I found myself an agent and did extra work for movies. I always wanted to model and act, but I wasn't tall enough or pretty enough for modelling. I entered a talent search contest back in my hometown, and I saw one of the judges look at the other judges and run her finger down her nose. Right then, I knew I was never going to be a model. I did, however, win a gold medal for acting. I memorized a Calvin Klein commercial in about twenty minutes while I was waiting in line for my turn, and I knew that I did well. I could feel it! I was very proud of myself for that gold medal. That was it, this was my calling. I would pursue acting in some way.

I took a little class at my agent's office for acting so that I would have some kind of credit on my resume. The instructor and I became friends, and he gifted me a copy of *The Silva Mind Control Method*. I still have that book today. In fact, I have two copies because I thought I lost it in a move a couple of years ago, so I bought another one because I go back and reread it now and again as a refresher.

That was when I was first introduced to the power of the subconscious mind. I read the book and learned how to go to my alpha level. The Silva method teaches you to picture the way you want things to happen like on a movie screen, so I gave it a try.

At the time, I was pregnant with my second child, so I envisioned a blonde, blue-eyed healthy baby boy on my screen. My husband has blue eyes and was blonde as a child, so it was entirely possible that our child could be born with his attributes.

Since this was my second child, I decided to find out the sex of the baby, and it was a boy. My blue-eyed, strawberry blonde-haired son is now an adult.

Is it coincidence? It could be, because of my husband's colouring, but our first child has my hazel green eyes and brown hair, and the mother usually has the dominant gene. Therefore, there was a fifty-fifty chance that our second child would have my colouring, too.

I believe that I manifested it. You can disagree with me, but I believe that this was my first experience with using the power of mind control.

After the birth of my son in 1998, I tried to keep practicing meditation when I went to bed at night. I would often fall asleep, which isn't a bad thing, but with two young children to care for, meditation fell to the wayside. At the time, I didn't think about using meditation to improve or create a better life. I was just absorbed in my life as the mom of two young children.

In the mid-2000s, my focus turned to the law of attraction and away from meditation because of where I was in my life. I was raising two young children and life was pretty good, so gratitude was working for me! It would be about fifteen years before I took up meditation again.

It wasn't until I was struggling to make sense of my life that I remembered what a valuable tool meditation could be. To be with oneself is calming.

It was 2023 before I started making all the connections. I was on the search for any, and all forms of positive reinforcement that I could find. It took me a while to put two and two together, but I wondered about a connection between Silva's mind control and the meditations we do today. Could there be a connection between them? During meditation, was I at the alpha level taught in mind control? Could I use both practices at the same time?

I started trying it. I pressed my thumb, index finger, and middle finger together on each hand as I lay in a comfortable position, generally in bed, after I first woke in the morning. This signaled my brain to enter the alpha level, as taught in Silva Mind Control. I learned how to do this way back when I first read the book, twenty-seven years before. I was enthused that the ability to reach alpha level had stayed with me, like riding a bike. After repeating this technique for a while, I was able to enter alpha quickly just by pressing my fingers together.

At the same time, I put headphones on and listened to a guided meditation. At first, I listened to everything out loud, but then learned I would have a better experience using headphones.

Sometimes I chose meditations on abundance and wealth. Other times I opted to work on my mindset or clearing blockages in my body. I selected a meditation on a topic that resonated with me at that moment. It varied between health, love, wealth, or bliss. Even manifesting my ideal reality. There are so, so many topics out there.

The alpha state is where I began and then ascended from there as I moved through the meditation. As I listened to the voice of the meditation guide, guru, or master manifester, whomever I selected that day, with my thumb and fingers touching, I told myself I was floating. I could feel my body getting lighter and lighter. As the meditation guided me deeper into the trance, I listened, visualized, and affirmed myself as prompted, all the time feeling like I was floating. It is then, at the calmest and freest state, that I was in tune with the law of vibration.

The law of vibration states that everything in the universe is in constant movement and is vibrating at a specific frequency. Another way to put it is that everything in motion, stays in motion. The higher one can vibrate, the higher the frequency. The higher the frequency, the more in tune with the universe one is.

This was the key I became aware of through meditation. It wasn't just about writing down what I was grateful for, it was about vibrating at the frequency that matched those things on my paper.

During meditation, as you picture your desires, you must be on the same frequency as that desire, or in other words, be in a state of vibration that matches what you are seeking to achieve. We are always in a state of vibration, but I understood that you need to vibrate at 500 HZ or more to be in frequency with the law of vibration. Some people come by it naturally, and others must work at it a little more, but when you get there, the world opens to the realm of possibilities.

Meditation provided me with my first opportunity to be in an altered state, and it was in that state that the magic began to happen.

I was free to think, dream and visualize in this state. There was nothing to fear and everything to create.

There are no limits to what we can do in this state. We create based on our level of consciousness. It is within our own state of consciousness and imagination that we create the path of our lives, including how our lives go during menopause.

The diagram below shows the levels of consciousness as they pertain to our feelings and the vibrational match to those feelings.

Omega

Level	Scale
Enlightenment	700+
Peace	600
Joy	540
Love	500
Reason	400
Acceptance	350
Willingness	310
Neutrality	250
Courage	200
Pride	175
Anger	150
Desire	125
Fear	100
Grief	75
Apathy	50
Guilt	30
Shame	20

Alpha

I had been vibrating so low for such a long time because I allowed myself to get caught up in all the negativity of everything I was going through. I was stuck in a victim mentality. I was wallowing, feeling caught in a vicious circle of uncertainty, going round and round without an end. I had forgotten that I had the power to make things better or worse at my disposal the whole time. I had the power in me to change how I felt at any time.

Once I implemented meditation daily, things started to improve. My entire attitude was changing. While I was in a calm, relaxed state, I was in a state of peace, which according to the chart vibrates at 600HZ. I pictured myself as I wanted to be. I told my body to be healthy and well. I commanded my hormones to balance and to be in perfect mental health. It was an art form.

I focused on the power I had within so that my external being would comply. I told my body it was healthy and well, and before long, it all started to happen! My hot flashes diminished in frequency and intensity. I had bloodwork done and my estrogen was on the rise and my cortisol was approaching normal levels. The frequent infections I had been suffering from ceased. I started sleeping again! I was starting to feel livelier and enjoying life again. My anger and resentment started to diminish, and I even wanted to engage in intimacy again.

As time went on, my life was becoming increasingly better, and I had the practice of meditation, and myself most of all, to thank. The changes I went through were internal, not external, going back to changing things in me to change things for me.

Now, meditation is part of my morning routine. My day doesn't feel the same if I can't do it right away or miss a morning. It has become an integral part of my life that provides me with a path to create my life the way I want it to be. It gives me the opportunity to take time out for myself, to work on myself, and to start my day in the proper mindset. I choose my mood. I choose what I am grateful for, and I choose my thoughts. I am in control!

My favourite meditations are:
Bob Proctor: Abundance Meditation
Bob Proctor: Shifting Your Paradigm
Regan Hillyer: Manifesting Your Ideal Reality
Paul McKenna: Hypnotic Trance for Bliss
Paul McKenna: Hypnotic Trance: Instant Confidence

*I am in tune
with my body's
needs and respond
with kindness*

CHAPTER THREE

Solfeggio Frequencies Are My Jam

I love solfeggio frequencies for healing my body, mind, and spirit. Not in a religious way, but in a positive, puts me in the right frame of mind kind of way.

I was drawn to seek out this music and I am so glad that I did! I knew about solfeggio frequencies, and I was looking for any and all means that I could find to bring me to a better place than where I was. I was on a mission to improve my mental health so that I could live a healthy, loving, fulfilling life even though I was in menopause.

I was in therapy again. I was also exercising and trying to eat better again, but my blood sugar made it very difficult to stay away from carbs, so I was frustrated with everything. I was reading inspiring material and writing down my gratitude list daily with the goal of feeling better, and at first it seemed like it was a very slow process.

I had been struggling for long enough. It was time. I was tired of feeling tired and tired of feeling depressed. I was tired of just existing in my life. I was tired of my body feeling unbalanced and my mental state along with it.

Solfeggio frequencies are an ancient musical scale of sorts. Each frequency taps into a specific part of the brain waves and the parasympathetic nervous system to initiate a response in either a mental or physical manner.

When I listen to a specific frequency, it raises my vibration, relieves stress, promotes calmness, reduces anxiety, and even initiates better quality sleep when I listen while in bed. Each frequency is in tune with my vibrational match and elevates my being, sometimes even creating a feeling of euphoria. I come away feeling positive, energized, and at my highest level of being.

Some examples of frequencies and how they can help you are:

174HZ: Concentration and pain relief
396HZ: Release guilt, fear, and anxiety
432HZ: Peace and wellbeing
528HZ: The love frequency
639HZ: Emotional balance
852HZ: In tune with your highest self
963HZ: Divine consciousness

I know it sounds like I was doing a lot, and for a while I was. I needed it. I was retraining my brain. All the positive affirmations, books, music, and gratitude lists are what helped me to begin my journey back to health.

I filled my waking hours with constant subjection to all that was positive. I played solfeggio music in the background while I worked and read inspirational books before bed.

Connection to this music brings me to a place of happiness and joy like nothing else I have done. It's my jam!

For me, it's the easiest way to raise my vibration, and when I raise my vibration, I become open to receiving. When I am open to receiving, I manifest and live the life I desire.

Let me meditate and listen to solfeggio frequencies, then look out world. I want it. I choose it. I live it. I am inspired and feel like I could change the world, and so it is!

*I found my frequencies on YouTube.

I am grateful
for the experiences
and lessons I have
learned during
menopause

CHAPTER FOUR

Discovering Gratitude In A New Way

I was introduced to *The Secret* and the power of gratitude in the mid-2000s, not long after the movie came out and I was enamoured with it. I welcomed new ways to live a better and happier life.

I gobbled it up as much as I could. I practiced and was grateful and I started to see positive changes happen in my life and around me. Wow! This stuff really works.

I watched the movie over and over a few times and bought the book. Truth be told, I bought a few of the pertaining books by some of the manifesters in the movie. I bought, *The Answer, The Vision Board, Life Lessons for Manifesting the Law of Attraction, The Key to Living the Law of Attraction,* and a few others. At that time in my life, I needed a positive escape. I thought my life would be fantastic once I had mastered all of these concepts.

When I first started applying the gratitude principles, I thought that just by saying that I was grateful for something that it would to come to fruition. Sure, Rhonda Byrne and the rest of the cast of the movie spoke of really feeling what you are grateful for, but how did I do that?

I know now that there were times when I was vibrating at the frequency to manifest what I wanted. But there were also times that I was not. It wasn't something that was coming to me naturally, or so I believed.

I was convinced I wasn't in tune with the frequency aspect of manifestation. Somewhere, I had missed that part of creating what you want. The law of vibration wasn't something that crossed my mind and I can see now, looking back, that had I clued into that, things would probably have been very different for me.

All the material I read only discussed the law of attraction. Be grateful and attract what you want was the message I understood. So, I did. I wrote down a list every day of things I was grateful for.

My husband was also on board with the law of attraction at the time. Between the two of us using the law, things were going really well, for a while, at least.

We had found a great friend group. My husband was doing well at work, the kids were growing and thriving, and I was rediscovering my voice again, literally. I had originally gone to university for music as a voice major but didn't end up finishing my degree. So, I found some guys on a musician's website, and we formed a band: Lisa and The Tallymen. Not the best name at all, I know, but the logic was that there were four other musicians and I was the lead singer, making the fifth. Our emblem was four lines with the fifth crossing through it, like when you are adding.

We were now able to afford to take the kids on family vacations. I felt very fortunate for the life we had, and we were creating it in our daily actions.

As time went on though, it seemed that the gratitude I was expressing wasn't having the same results that it once did. It seemed hard to keep it all up. My husband kind of fell off the wagon as he got busier with his career and raising the kids. I kept at it, but it didn't seem to have the same effect and I didn't know why, but now I understand that I wasn't evolving in the material. I had been doing the same thing for years without learning anything new.

Amid all this, I forgot that life still happens, and we were faced with a family crisis that involved one of our children. At that time, being grateful was the last thing I was. I had to focus on taking care of my family. I remember thinking: how can I be grateful right now?

Feelings of hurt, pain, and resentment were a part of my reality for a time, but I mustered through, making sure those who needed protection were protected. For many years, I believed that I was being punished for something I, or we, had done. We all do stupid things when we are young and trying to figure out who we are, and we were no different. We were being taught a lesson because of our own selfish behaviours. God couldn't be that cruel, could he?

We had to examine our lives and reevaluate our priorities. When bad things happen, people look for ways to cope and get through it. Some choose religion, others go to therapy, and there are those who turn to self-medicating to numb the pain. I have tried religion and therapy in the past, but for me, immersing myself in positive affirmations makes me feel better than praying to God or talking to any therapist.

Don't get me wrong, I believe in a higher power that could be called 'God,' but my head was in a space that didn't like God very much at that moment in time. I was hurt and in pain, which clouded my state of mind. I was after something different than the same old routine.

I think that maybe God provided the opportunity that would lead me down a path that I needed to be on. I had spent years unhappily going to church and praying. Could God be guiding me to expand my mind into the realm of possibilities? Could God be showing me that I could have more out of life? Could God want me to be happy?

When I was younger, if you asked me if I was happy, I would have answered, "What is happiness anyway?" That answer was from a person who always looked outside herself to find happiness. She thought happiness came in the form of other people or circumstances, not within herself. She had no clue how to really be happy. She was playing the role of life instead of living it.

The universal laws have taken me to a place that has inspired concrete values, opening a new side of me that had been hidden away for a long time. It was a time of rebirth and renewal for me. I experienced a personal cleansing of my inner being that made me feel so much better about myself and my life than any counsellor ever did. I had come a long way. I had rediscovered gratitude in a whole new way that was transformative on many levels. For once, I felt like I knew what it was like to be happy, and it felt great!

*I am beautiful
and I am thriving
during menopause!*

CHAPTER FIVE

Using Affirmations and Lucky Girl Syndrome

It was such an important step to move forward freely, but to do so, I had to look back, into my past. How did I grow up? How did I feel about myself when I was younger? What experiences shaped who I am now?

I was a child of the 70s. We didn't wear bike helmets or seatbelts. We stayed out until the streetlights came on and foods like ketchup and cheese in jars didn't have expiry dates.

Growing up, I struggled with self-confidence. It would be easy to place blame on my parents, to say that I didn't receive the encouragement or support I needed. Maybe that's true, but I don't hold them responsible. I was loved in the way they knew how to love, and I recognize that my parents did their best, especially with seven mouths to feed. I say 'knew how' because the era in which they were raised was different. Both came from large families themselves, and they were the only ones on either side to have more than three children.

No one read them stories or tucked them in at night. They shared bedrooms with two, three, or even four siblings. They started work at a young age and didn't finish high school, let alone go to college.

But I admired them. After we had all moved out and were married, the family would go back to Mom and Dad's for barbecues. Sometimes after dinner, we would go for a walk to the water to see the boats. When

I grew up there was an amusement park on an island called Bob-Lo Island. It attracted boaters and the like because you could only get to the island two ways: by ferry from my hometown in Canada, or by riverboat from Detroit, Michigan. On these occasions, my parents walked hand in hand, and I knew I wanted that for myself one day. They loved each other, even when things weren't easy. Sure, they had their fair share of disagreements, but at no time did I ever think they would not be together.

I was bullied a lot as a child and had only a few friends. 'Bullied' wasn't a term in the seventies when I grew up. We called it 'teasing,' but it's the same thing. I was teased from grade four to eight, which is why I went to a totally different high school than everyone else. Things were different back then. Teachers didn't pay attention to things like kids being bullied. If they did notice, most of the time, nothing was ever done about it. Once I graduated from grade eight, I wanted to get away from all my abusers, so I chose to go to a high school that was an hour bus ride away. It was the best thing I ever did for myself!

I was made to feel like I wasn't good enough by both boys and girls for a very long time. I didn't feel pretty or smart enough. I didn't live at the right end of town. I didn't wear the skintight pants or have the latest fashions; I had a lot of hand me downs. Since I was the youngest of so many, my parents weren't as young and 'cool' like some of the other parents. I was also born with astigmatism so my eyes twitched. I just felt different from everyone else and spent way too much time alone with my own thoughts.

I remember trying to act confidently. I tried so hard not to let the teasing bother me, but of course, it did. I was alone a lot of the time at home because my siblings were so much older than me. The oldest married when I was nine. The next was when I was thirteen. Then three more siblings' weddings the year I turned seventeen, which was 1985. After that, I was the only one left at home with Mom and Dad for the next six years.

At school, kids decided to tease me about some stupid thing one boy said he saw. He claimed he saw me picking my nose, so I became Lisa Rose Picks Her Nose. I can't even remember if it was true, but I remember how I was treated. Don't ask me why everyone believed him or ran with it, but they did, and then it was decided that I was an outcast.

It was difficult for me and made me sensitive to some behaviours from others. I was an overthinker, even back then. I would spend hours thinking about what was so bad about me. To get myself through the day, I told myself that bullies had their own issues at home and that is why they bullied.

I was raised Roman Catholic and was a regular churchgoer. I went to a Catholic grade school and high school (high school was my choice). I joined a religious group while at university. I believed in God and took the body and blood of Christ at services. I also sang in the Church choir and remained a virgin until I was twenty because that is what I thought I should do as a good Catholic girl.

I also went through a phase where I thought of becoming a nun. I was religious and, like many teens, I had no idea what I was going to do with my life.

One thing was for certain: when bad things have happened in my life, I always believed that God was punishing me for something; a choice I had made or didn't make. If my life was too good for a while, I was due for some family trauma or a life-altering challenge to have to deal with.

It felt like other girls were always prettier. The boys I liked didn't like me back, and those that did like me, weren't my taste at all. I felt bad about myself and wondered what was wrong with me. When I looked in the mirror, I thought I was cute! I certainly didn't think I was any less pretty than my friends. I was a nice person as well, yet, they had boyfriends, and I didn't. Maybe some were putting out, I don't know. If I had met the right person, I may not have waited until I was twenty, either. Who knows?

Even though I didn't feel adequate a lot of the time, I always had this thought that someday I would do great things with my life. I was going to be a successful singer, actor, model, or something. I have never been shy of the limelight. Maybe I have something to prove to all those who teased me during grade school and hurt me in high school. I required accreditation and validation to make me feel good about myself. When I say something intelligently, I want the acknowledgement that I am 'smartacle', as I call it in my house.

Now, I can clearly see, that I was living from a victim mentality. I always just let things happen to me instead of creating things for me. On occasion I found the guts to speak up for what I wanted, but when I did, often, I was disappointed with the results. Looking back, I lived in a bubble of complete naivety.

I was lonely, and on a quest to find love. I wanted to be with someone, like my friends were. I was searching for companionship on an intimate level, even for a little while. I longed to be hugged and held. I was hoping for someone to hold my hand and to talk to. I wished for someone who I liked, to like me back as more than a friend.

In my pursuit to happiness, I think I've had some interesting men come and go from my life, but there were a couple that stood out as particularly unique to me. Since I am an overthinker, I used to wonder what it was about me, that drew this kind of attention from these guys. I wanted to know, because for a long time, I blamed God for not bringing me love.

My husband says I have 'kavorka', like from the 90's TV show, Seinfeld. According to the urban dictionary, 'kavorka' (pronounced kah-vor-kah), means 'the lure of the animal', making someone irresistible, especially those of a different sex. That would explain some things, but then again, I was a girl who thought about becoming a nun, so having sexual energy was the last thing I would have thought I possessed.

In the first semester of my first year of university, there was a guy, let's call him John, who I met through a mutual acquaintance. John seemed nice and we were kind of friends. We both attended an overnight religious retreat, where John tried to get me to have sex with him. It took me by surprise considering where we were at the time.

During the night's events, we sang songs and praised God like good worshippers do. Afterward, we all retired to our rooms to call it a night, but it wasn't long before there was a knock at my door. It was him, my 'friend' John, so I let him in.

We chatted for a couple of minutes, but then John leaned forward and started kissing me. I was eighteen by this time, so I had some experience in this area and knew that people 'hooked up' but I was hesitant to reciprocate. I generally didn't just 'hook up', after all, I had considered becoming a nun just a few short years prior. It all felt very uncomfortable, especially when John tried to take it to the bed, asking to do the deed right there and then. I thought, Wow! Really! At a religious function? It was not only blasphemy but seemed pretty desperate.

Call me a goodie-two-shoes, but when you're not ready, you're not ready. I wasn't the kind of girl who slept around. I was looking for a relationship, so I kicked John to the curb and that 'friendship' was over as fast as it began.

During my second semester, which would have been after Christmas 1987, there was a guy who wrote me anonymous letters. I'll call him Jake. Jake wrote me, saying that he thought I was the most attractive girl he had ever seen. Who? Me?

I wondered who was playing this joke on me. It was no joke. Jake wrote me three or four letters in total before he let himself be known. He was having a mutual friend post the letters to the message board in the hall of the music building, where I had most of my classes. As I walked by going from room to room, I saw my name handwritten on a folded piece of paper, which was stuck to the cork board with a thumb tack.

After I received a couple of letters, I went into the room and asked out loud, 'Who's playing this joke on me?' Who was this? I asked myself as I glanced around the music school common room, examining every person. Hearing what I said, the mutual friend told Jake I thought the letters were a cruel joke, so he finally revealed himself.

I was surprised when I found out who Jake was. We had only met once at a rehearsal between the university school of music and the city symphony. On occasion, the two performed together and as part of the music program, I was required to sing in the University Choir. It was the Christmas of 1987 and together, the choir and the symphony performed a beautiful rendition of the Hallelujah Chorus.

I was nineteen and Jake was twenty-seven. He was tall, around six feet, and had auburn hair. While chatting, we each shared where we were from, and to our surprise, we lived in the same town. Cool! That would make seeing each other easy.

He also had his own car since he was done with school a few years earlier and playing in the symphony was his job. Jake was the first guy I dated who was done with school, had a job, and had his own car. I was really moving up!

When I asked him why he wrote me the letters, he said that he just wanted to. I think he was trying to be romantic, but I wasn't used to that kind of flattery and didn't know how to accept it.

After all the effort, Jake and I dated for a couple of months and then it fizzled out. We came in hot, so there was nowhere to go but down. We were at different phases of life; therefore, the age gap was also a factor.

Before John, the jerk and Jake the letter guy, going back to my high school years, there was someone who came into my life in an interesting way. He will be, Jonah. Jonah was someone who I had met through the school band, and we became friends. He was friendly, kind and overall, a nice guy.

Jonah was in grade twelve at the time and had been elected the band president, so he decided to have a band party at his house. I was fifteen, naïve and impressionable. I was caught off guard while walking down the hall to the bathroom, when out of nowhere, Jonah pulled me into a bedroom. Before I could say anything, he began to kiss me. Looking to be loved, I kissed him back, and I liked it. From the limited experience I had at that point, I thought he was a great kisser.

Being a grade niner, I thought, Oh wow, Jonah must like me. Like in a romantic way. I was wrong. He never treated me the same afterward and I never understood why. Maybe he was embarrassed, I don't know. Jonah had been my friend, so it never crossed my mind, that sometimes people make out at parties and then move on with life.

Welcome to high school! It was kicked off with its share of teenage drama.

This story doesn't quite end here, there's more. That was grade nine and the first time Jonah and I had an encounter at a band party. The next year, when I was in grade ten, there was another party. I know what you're thinking, and yes, I did. I was young and vulnerable.

The second time was on me. I should have known better, but I was still trying to mend fences from the year before. Since I struggled with confidence in myself, I was trying to figure out what I had done wrong to make Jonah ignore me the way he did. I didn't understand why we couldn't still be friends.

Somehow, we found ourselves in Jonah's room. The next thing I knew, we were locking lips heatedly, and I was whisked into the closet. My common sense was telling me I shouldn't be there, engaging with Jonah like this again. My sixteen-year-old hormones were saying something very different. He was such a good kisser, I couldn't resist.

Then it happened. Jonah asked me the big question. Out of sight, hiding in the cramped, dark, clothes-cluttered closet, he asked me to be his first. What? I was sixteen and inexperienced in that way, so I quickly and awkwardly declined, (though there have been times I wonder what would have happened if I said yes). Lots of girls start having sex at sixteen.

Thinking back on it now, I feel flattered that he chose me to ask me to be his first, whether I was just the girl who was at the right place at the right time, or not.

Forty years ago, that sixteen-year-old inexperienced girl was wounded. Again, Jonah wouldn't speak to her after the party, and she wondered how someone who was going to serve God, could treat her the way he did. Maybe he just didn't know what to say. It could be a guy thing. Notch in the belt, or whatever.

When he graduated, Jonah went off to the seminary to become a Catholic priest, so I can see why he would want to experience what sex was like before he gave it up for the rest of his life. I didn't understand that then, of course. I had no idea what was going on in Jonah's head.

I can't explain why I was so fascinated with Jonah. I just wanted to be loved by someone, and for a minute I thought it could be him. For a minute, in that dark, cramped closet, I thought I felt the connection I was looking for. But alas, I was disappointed.

It was shortly after that experience, I thought that maybe I should become a nun. I was so confused. After the close encounter with the closet, I thought, What the hell, God?! Why are you doing this to me? What do you want from me? Don't I deserve to be loved by someone? Left with a lasting impression, once Jonah was gone from my everyday school life, I eventually moved on, with what seemed like, no help from God. In my case, I had no choice; he was in the seminary, on his way to give his life to God.

Years later, when I was twenty-three, I ran into Jonah, and we actually had a conversation without any making out involved. In case you're curious, no, he did not end up becoming a priest.

The summer I turned twenty, I finally did find the kind of love I longed for. The stars had aligned, and it seemed like we had been destined to be together. We both worked at the local Burger King and met each other through mutual friends. By this time, after my previous experiences, I knew what I was looking for in a partner. I wanted to be with someone who was compassionate, kind, loving, honest and made me feel special. This guy had a life plan and wanted the same things I did from it.

I had no idea at the time, but he liked me for about six months before he asked me out on our first date. I was seeing Jake, anonymous letter guy, and found out later, that the man who became my future husband had waited patiently until I was free.

His parents were divorced, and his father was getting remarried, so he asked me to the wedding. His dad's wedding was our first date. A wedding first date. No pressure.

Right away, I liked being with him and he was the kind of person who was easy to get along with. I was comfortable with him and could talk to him about almost anything. He made me feel safe when no one else ever did. He was easy to love, but most importantly, he loved me just the way I was, hangups and all.

He had the deepest blue eyes I had ever seen, and I was lost in them easily when I stared into them. He was considerate, funny and intelligent. I thought, Wow, this guy is the one. I've found my soulmate.

He kissed me good night when he brought me home from the wedding and I felt a flutter in my stomach that I had not felt before.

That was June 18, 1988, and we have been together since. Like many long-term relationships, it hasn't been without its own challenges, but as of September 2024 we will have been together for thirty-six years and married thirty-three. He tells me I'm beautiful and we still have a loving, supportive life together. We have raised a great family and I'm so very proud of that. I still get that flutter in my stomach when he kisses me.

Sometimes my inner voice would tell me I wasn't worthy of a good life though, and it was her I listened to the most. She was practical. She was a wife, mother, and had lots of jobs, but never a career.

I started to find some confidence as I got a little older. I think my early thirties were my best years. I was done having children and they were out of diapers. I was thin and started colouring my hair red, which made my hazel green eyes pop! I looked good and I felt more confident about myself. My marriage was going well. We had a great friend group, a comfortable home, and were doing reasonably well financially.

I had missed out on a lot of fun kid stuff as a young girl and as a teenager. I finally had friends as a teen and was even part of the school band, but I never had someone to love in my personal life the way I longed to be loved until much later. When I went home from school, I was alone.

Years passed before I was introduced to 'I AM' statements and started repeating them. Many times, I was brought to tears. I still get choked up now and again.

It has taken a long time for me to say and believe statements like, 'I am beautiful,' 'I am loved,' and 'I am worthy of abundance.' Sure, I could say the words easily enough, but did I believe them?

Belief in yourself is up there with loving yourself, so this was difficult to get used to. I could be grateful all day long but believing that I was worthy of success and love was another story. Hence me saying, 'If I can do this, so can you!'

I had to decide that I wanted a better life for myself, so one day I thought, Why not give it a try? I started to repeat positive affirmations to myself as much as I could. I kept at it daily. I practiced and practiced.

I read *The Secret to Love, Health, and Money: A Masterclass* and *The Magic* by Rhonda Byrne. Paired with the affirmations, these two books were a big part of the change I could feel happening in me.

Before long I wasn't just reading or listening to positive affirmations, I was writing my own as part of my daily gratitude practice.

I am kind. I am gracious. I am patient. I am understanding. I am in good health. I am strong. I am powerful. What, I am powerful? Yes! You better believe you are!

I am in charge of my life. I am in a loving, caring relationship with the best person for me. I am abundant. I am, I am, I am.

Then I started evolving my affirmations to be about specific topics, like my business: I am good at my job. I am creative. I am respected by my colleagues. I am deserving of success in everything I do.

Now I was getting bold! I am magnificent. I am fantastic. I am awesome.

Then it occurred to me: Why not say and write positive 'I AM' statements about menopause symptoms?

'I am having the best menopause journey.'
'I am in perfect health and my hormones are perfectly balanced.'
'I am so grateful for this wonderful time in my life.'
'I am so very grateful to be free of monthly cycles.'
'I am not alone in my experience.'
'I am experiencing the best time of my life.'
'I am sleeping soundly every night.'

I'm sure you get the idea. Now you try:

Write three 'I AM' statements about your menopause journey below. Be as specific as possible. The more specific you are, the better results you will have.

1. ____

    ____

    ____

2. ____

    ____

    ____

3. ____

    ____

    ____

Now repeat them back slowly and try to pay attention to your feelings about each statement. Are you going through the motions of the exercise, or do you really mean what you wrote?

If you answered the latter, do you feel any different? Repeat this for a few days in a row, then think of three different 'I AM' statements each day afterward. Note if you feel any different in general after each time you do this. It took me some time to understand what it means to 'feel it.'

You might think, 'What do you mean? I wrote it down so that should mean I feel it!' Not necessarily. Feeling is believing and believing is feeling, so if you truly believe in what you wrote down, you will feel something happening inside. It's similar to a feeling of excitement. That's how you know the magic is happening.

'I AM statements gave me the opportunity to put what I am grateful for in different words. They were powerful proclamations that hyped me up, got my juices flowing, and reinforced that I am just as worthy as everyone else to have all that life has to offer. Positive affirmations coincide with having a good attitude. It's all mindset and mine was improving.

'I AM' statements are now the little voice in my head telling me I am worthy; I am just as important as other people, and I am deserving of success.

I don't stop there, though. I affirm myself with statements like:

'I have all the tools I need to overcome my challenges and achieve my goals.'

'My worth is inherent, and I deserve to be treated with kindness and compassion.'

'Every day brings new opportunities to learn and become a better version of myself.'

'My unique talents and qualities contribute to my success and make me valuable in my own unique way.'

'I control my thoughts and I choose to foster positivity and hope in my life

'Menopause is liberating, and I love where I am in my life now.'

'Menopause is a beautiful phase of life.'

Lucky Girl Syndrome

What the hell is Lucky Girl Syndrome? Is it contagious? Will I catch it? I hope it is contagious! I am a lucky girl and so is every other meno-pausal woman!

Lucky girl syndrome (LGS) is a movement. It is a manifestation thought process that uses the law of assumption. The law of assumption suggests that by believing something has already happened, it will manifest itself.

LGS was adopted by various social media users and suggests implementing positive life habits to bring about good luck. It pro-motes having an optimistic outlook, using affirmations, creating self-belief, the power of manifestation, and the practice of gratitude.

I discovered LGS while searching for something else on YouTube in early 2024. I caught a few lines and was hooked! Positive affirma-tions. Manifestation. Gratitude. This was right up my alley! Where do I sign up?

The concept is based on knowing that everything will work out in your favour. Yes, please!

Some examples are:

'Everything is always working out for me.'

'Amazing opportunities are coming my way today.'

'I am deserving of an abundant life.'

'I am the luckiest person I know.'

'People want to do things for me.'

'I am beautiful inside and out.

'Everything I desire comes to me easily.'

'I only attract good things.'

Subliminal messaging? If I listened to LGS affirmations while falling asleep, I would wake in a better mood and have better luck. Sounded good to me!

Like the other tools I adopted, when I listened to Lucky Girl Syndrome affirmations, I could feel my vibration rising. My heart started beating faster, my blood pressure elevated, and I felt this rush of greatness come over me. I thought, Yes, I am invincible! Look out world!

This was the emotional state of being I wanted to stay in. This was a feeling that gave me energy to combat my demons. This was the highest of high vibrations, where I was able to solidify my desires in stone.

I was using these various techniques simultaneously because that's what I wanted to do. I wanted to experience as much as I could to create and embrace my desired outcome, which was peace and harmony within myself. Each meditation, each frequency, each visualization were all connected. One dot led to the next, and then the next.

It was important to me, my growth, and my mindset, so I made the time. I found time in the morning, at night and while I was working. I listened to what brought me up in copious amounts to maintain a high vibrational state.

I was growing and evolving. My mindset was shifting, and I wanted more. Repetition creates habit and I was repeating, absorbing, and living what I exposed myself to. I had faith in myself and the process I was undertaking. I was on a high and I loved it all! I was creating. I was the creator.

The higher I vibrated, the happier I felt. The more I visualized myself in my desired life, the happier I felt. The happier I felt, the more my life aligned. The more my life aligned, the easier menopause became. It was a true definition of the trickle effect. One good thought led to another, then another and another.

Give me my affirmations, my solfeggio frequencies, and my meditation. Give me my gratitude journal and my community. Give me my high-vibrational state and my imagination and I will give you an extremely lucky girl!

Each day,

I grow stronger

and more resilient

during menopause

CHAPTER SIX

Setbacks and Triggers

Just when I thought I was embracing my new way of life, out of nowhere it would happen. I went from feeling invincible to crying for the entire day. What a whirlwind of emotions to try to handle!

I have had some definite setbacks on my mindset journey. There were some days where I questioned the process and whether all that I was doing was really making an impact.

Some days I woke up and didn't have it in me to be happy or thankful and mean it. Some days it was all I could do to get out of bed, clean myself, and start work. Some days felt like the universe was working against me. Some days I questioned my entire life. Some days I was discouraged. Some days I wanted to chuck it in because I was having so much trouble resonating at the right vibration.

Some days I took a break, and it was okay; I survived. There were some days when I just didn't think about anything, good or bad. I just wanted to exist for a moment or two to just be quiet with myself and block out the world.

I found that being still and quiet with myself and relaxing in my way, re-energized me. I liked to watch movies, take a bath, be near water, meditate, or read and just be alone. No demands on me. No pressures. Just me.

Maybe my need to be alone goes back to my childhood when I spent so much time in my own company. I do what I want to do without the input from anyone else. I just try not to talk to myself too much (haha).

There have been a few times when a setback and a trigger episode were combined. Every doubt I ever had about myself was back. Those were tough days. They lasted for a day or two, until I sorted out my inner work. In some cases, when I was triggered, it would cause a setback with my self-work. Then, when ready, I picked myself up and began again.

I didn't want to give up. I had given up on myself too many times before and I deserved better. I was determined to see this work to the end this time; to see me as I want to see myself. I was determined to tell myself that I could do this. I could shed the fear, pain, and every other negative feeling that had been plaguing me for far too long.

There are some people who don't like the word 'triggered,' but I feel the word describes how it was for me when I felt everything in my life was out of control.

According to Dr. David Richo, in the book, *How We Can Stop Reacting and Start Healing Triggers*, 'A trigger is any word, person, event, or experience that touches off an immediate emotional reaction, especially sadness/depression, anger/aggression, fear/panic, or humiliation/shame.'

After I read the definition in that book, I finally understood what it was I experienced when in situations that made me uncomfortable. I just wanted to run away from whatever was happening at the time until either I gathered myself or the situation passed. There were even times I would avoid social settings because I didn't want to put myself out there. I was fearful of being judged by everyone, including family, so I even avoided some family gatherings.

I thought I knew what all my triggers were. They were specific in nature and most of them revolved around my personal relationship with sex during menopause.

I was stressed to the max on that topic, so any mention of being sexy, looking sexy, or engaging in anything out of the ordinary during sex, I retreated into myself and put-up walls that were higher than the Great Wall of China! I was impenetrable, both literally and figuratively.

I had a few instances where I was caught completely off guard by a triggering situation. My body started to tremble and go into a cold sweat, feeling completely beside myself. I was triggered for reasons unknown that caused my body to switch off and shut down. I couldn't leave or run away so I became very quiet. Some might say I was rude, but that's what I needed to do to gather myself. I felt this rush of fight or flight happening inside my belly and I began to feel nervous and anxious. Any decorum of social etiquette went out the window. I could do nothing but sit quietly and wait until the feelings passed, then I could function like a human again. I just wanted to be left alone. I didn't want anyone to talk to me, I just wanted them to leave me be. I was so embarrassed after each of these instances, and I know it has affected some relationships.

It's difficult to recover socially after an instance like that. I didn't want to discuss my personal situation, nor could I really explain what was going on with me without sounding like a crazy woman, so I thought the best course was to move on and not talk about what happened to anyone unless they brought it up first. The opinion I took was that everyone has bad days, so I was allowed to have them, too. I mean really, did I hurt anyone? No. Did I endanger anyone? No. I just embarrassed myself and I had to live with that.

Learning to recognize and handle my triggers has been a journey in and of itself. When you react a certain way for a long period of time, it becomes almost second nature, so I have worked very hard at retraining my brain. I've learned a lot about fear and where it stems from, so I now understand that most of my triggers come from fear. Fear causes me anxiety and sleeplessness. Fear causes me undue stress. Fear builds my walls and drains my energy.

I have sought out counselling several times over the years, and I have found it to be a big help to unload my shit onto someone who was unbiased. It's like a weight being lifted off my shoulders to be able to share my burdens with someone who isn't judging me.

I had reached a point where I was becoming seriously concerned about my mental health, so I decided to be evaluated by a psychiatrist. I wanted to know if there was something medically wrong with me, or if all this craziness was just part of my menopause life.

I have a family history of mental illness, so I wanted to be sure about what was going on in my head. Whether or not it was just menopause related, the psychiatrist diagnosed me with clinical depression and PTSD. What? PTSD! That was something I hadn't thought about. Depression, yes, but post-traumatic stress disorder came as a surprise.

I had to decide where to go from there. Should I obsess over this diagnosis from one doctor who was practically falling asleep in my session? Should I get a second opinion? Or should I fight? Should I take it with a grain of salt and just work on being more mindful of myself, my actions, and my persona?

I would have to learn to take all the negative emotions, fears, and anxiety, along with guilt, and turn it into thinking in a positive way about my life, including what I thought of myself. I have felt a lot of guilt, and it is hard to let go of it. There are just some things that, no matter how hard you try, stay with you, even if in a small way.

Though it's said that time does not exist, the process didn't happen overnight. It has taken me a year of focusing on what has been going on inside me. The setbacks I experienced due to my triggers began to allow me to self-reflect and adjust my thought process. In that respect, they have been a learning tool for my path forward. They have given me more ammunition to work and grow with, but there are days when it is difficult for me to move forward. I can be hard on myself to just get over it, but setbacks are a part of life. I can be impatient with myself, so I must keep in mind that shit happens, and life goes on.

Circumstances don't have to be dramatic and life-changing. I don't have to wallow in self-pity. Instead, I can feel the feels (that's important) and then move on. I'm not saying I'm perfect at it. Moving on from some things is still a work in progress, but I feel optimistic that I am moving in the right direction.

If everything happens for a reason, then I should be the f-ing luckiest girl on the planet by now! Some days I can't comprehend the reason why things happen. Then I hear the little voice in my head reminding me that I am creating whatever is happening with me myself. Sometimes I must go through the bad to get to the good, then keep going to make the good great.

So, the setbacks I experienced have been an opportunity to think better thoughts and let go of the past. Be a better human. Be clear about what I want and set a plan in motion to make it all happen.

They give me the chance to take a moment to breathe and reflect on the situation at hand; the chance to think in that moment of my next action. They provide a gateway to keep working and moving forward. To keep progressing. To continue to retrain my brain to handle anything that comes my way.

I would have never thought I would be grateful for the challenging times I've experienced, but I have come to know that great growth comes through the darkest of times.

My worth is not
defined by my age
or physical changes,
it is everlasting

CHAPTER SEVEN

Finding My Community

The best thing I did for myself was to find my community; other people who thought the way I did and believed in the power of mindset as I did.

I needed something. I needed to know I wasn't alone. I needed to talk to other people like me. I needed some outside opinions, so I searched Facebook for menopause support groups. Then I searched Instagram and TikTok, as well, for other women in menopause.

I found a couple of menopause support groups, so I joined them, thinking I would find support, which I did, but not in the way I was expecting.

Most of the time, women were posting all the things that sucked about menopause and the symptoms that go along with it. I was surprised to see some women talk about not showering or getting dressed for a couple of days. A couple spoke of getting rid of their husbands because they had no desire for sex. Admittedly, there was a time when I considered the same, but I always believed that it wasn't forever, and it should get better. Right? It was eye-opening to read what other women were going through, as well.

The more I read these posts, the more I found myself wanting to offer advice to help them feel better. There were some women who I shared similar woes with, but the more I read how difficult it had been for others, the more I didn't think of my own situation, I just wanted to help them.

I remember thinking that it was an interesting perspective because when I first thought about sharing my story, I was going to talk about how awful my journey was and that was it. My early blogs and TikTok videos tell that story, too. The me of only a couple of years ago felt the same way these women did and so I understood what they were going through. She was looking for others to wallow and complain with, and she was in the right place. She had found them.

The following quotes are examples of comments that people shared:

'I just want to sleep, and stop being hot and sweaty. I hate this shit. Five years in and I am tired.'

'I'm so sick of this weight gain. I don't know what to do!! I eat, I gain. I don't eat, I gain. I smell or look at food and I gain.'

'Every day, I try to hold in the tears. I feel horrible. My hair is falling out, I have anxiety, irritability, fear, depression, health anxiety. It's a lot to deal with daily.'

'Another thing to hate about menopause, it makes you want to cry about the littlest problems.'

'One year in real bad menopause, with no sign of light at the end of the tunnel. As soon as I take care of the symptoms, which seem to change every minute, a new one pops up.'

'I CAN'T deal with the anxiety / panic attacks. I overthink now so much! THIS ISN'T ME!'

As time went on, the Facebook groups lost their lustre. The more I was on the page, the more I found it was draining my energy to read the posts. Maybe these groups weren't what I was looking for after all. Maybe they weren't the kind of group I needed to belong to. I discovered that instead of complaining, I found myself wanting to be inspired and supported. While these groups offered support, it turned out that most of them were run by businesses affiliated with helping women with menopause. Every so often you would see a plug from the organization or counsellor that was moderating the group. Sigh.

I felt stagnated by the group. I was beginning to see that I had evolved past this kind of group. The inner work I was doing was paying off. I noticed more and more that I was asking women if they tried meditation or wrote in a journal. I asked if there was anyone who was thinking any good thoughts about their journey, or if there was anyone who was experiencing anything that was good about menopause. Were they happy to be rid of a monthly cycle? Did anyone think that their body was beautiful and healthy? What did women tell themselves?

I found myself wanting to help, but not on a Facebook page. I felt it should be bigger than that. It was like an intuition. So, I turned my attention to other media streams to see what else was out there and noticed a common theme among many of the menopause experts, naturopaths, and doctors. Everyone was either selling some sort of magic powder, potion, or supplement, and doctors recommended HRT (hormone replacement therapy) as the most effective way to treat menopausal symptoms. There were also people (because it wasn't only women, I saw some men) promoting one concoction or another that was sure to help you feel better.

While I am a believer in nourishing your body, and that exercise is a must during menopause, all I saw was several external remedies to alleviate symptoms. I'm not saying that you should not take supplements. I have my own supplements that I take to help produce estrogen and promote healthy bones, like vitamin D, vitamin E, and chasteberry. I also include collagen in my protein shakes.

Let's not forget the fitness gurus, spouting that one diet or another would be the cure-all for menopause symptoms. Don't eat carbs. Don't eat vegetables. Eat keto. Eat carnivore. Eat a balanced diet that includes vegetables and carbs. Which is it? Make up your mind.

I came to the conclusion that one size doesn't fit all. Every 'body' is different, you just have to find what fits yours. For the longest time, I couldn't stop craving carbs, but I finally found a balance that worked for me. Once I began to focus on being healthy, my body responded.

Few of the 'experts' spoke of the mindset to focus on symptoms. Some spoke of mindset, yes, not but in the way I was experiencing it. I was undergoing a mindshift in a different way, and I found myself wanting to help women do the same. I wanted to help women understand that they had the power within themselves to improve their symptoms by changing the way they thought about them. Attitude IS everything, as it turns out.

There is general mindset, but what I was going through was different than that. I moved past generality and focused on a specific area of my life. In this case it was my menopause symptoms, because that's what I chose to focus my attention on. It was the biggest thing going on in my life and it was the biggest thing affecting my quality of life.

One day, I was scrolling Instagram and saw that Shantelle Bisson, author of the Without Losing Your Cool book series, was promoting a guest on her podcast. Shantelle, whom I follow and have met, featured a guest who spoke about manifesting the life you want. I thought that it looked interesting, so I watched it. The guest was Kathleen Cameron. Kathleen completed Bob Proctor's program and has grown her coaching business exponentially in a short period of time.

Her message resonated with me in a big way, so I began to follow her on Instagram and looked up her group on Facebook. She had created a community page, so I requested to join. I had found it! This was the kind of group that I was looking for. I was amongst like-minded people who supported, encouraged, and uplifted one another.

Thank you, thank you, thank you! I was HOM (stands for House of Manifestation). I found my like-minded people and I was on my way to solidifying my beliefs, growing in my mindshift journey, and learning new tools that would assist me in moving forward. I was ascending faster and with more clarity.

Now, I focus my attention on creating my own space for growth and discovering the best ways to help other women take back their lives, as I did. I am supported the way I was looking to be in a group of people who think like me. I go to events that uplift and reestablish the gifts I possess and give to the world.

I drop in now and again to the former groups I was in to offer some words of encouragement to those who are suffering, like I was. My purpose there now is to let the women in the group know that I was there too, and that there is hope.

The tone of my social accounts and blogs has changed to focus on something I have learned or a positive message instead of complaining about things I cannot change. I feel more energized about myself and my life than I think I ever have. My outlook on everything has changed and feels right. It feels good, and I believe I am just getting started.

*I accept this phase
of my life with
confidence and grace*

CHAPTER EIGHT

Living the Menopause Mindshift

I was on a mission to be healthy. Therefore, I sought out various opinions to which path I should take to get there. More therapy? Medication? Cognitive Behaviour Therapy?

I wanted my menopause symptoms to cease, and I was getting there. I began sleeping better, my hot flashes improved, and even the electric shock feelings became few and far between.

My mindset was the key factor in my transformation, and I could sense it. Mindful eating and exercise were only a portion of the journey. The big changes came about when I put my mind to it . . . literally! When everything was working in sync, I saw faster results than implementing just one healthy habit.

The introduction to living life with a better attitude about menopause shifted my entire experience. My brain was going through a rewire. I was putting my own version of Cognitive Behaviour Therapy into effect. I had relived my past enough and was ready to put it behind me for good. I always could; I only had to choose to do it. I had to conjure up the strength to let it all go and keep moving forward.

Yes, I implemented many techniques, but it's been a wonderful adventure learning so much about myself and how I tick. I see now that I was going through life with blinders on. I wasn't living truly and meaningfully by letting the outside world influence how I felt. I wasn't in control of myself, and as a result my life was in chaos.

I allowed myself to be depressed. I allowed myself to be angry and I allowed myself to let other people dictate my feelings. The period of not giving a damn was over! I was retraining my own brain.

By definition, retraining the brain involves repetitious cognitive activity over a set period of time. The repetition creates new neural connections that form a desired outcome or behaviour. In other words, repetition creates habit. In my case, I wanted to make my life better as a whole, but I wanted it to begin with my menopause symptoms.

I had the knowledge I needed from the books and various mental activities I was pursuing. I had the tools available to put a plan in place. I simply had to decide to start.

I took the first step by identifying my negative thoughts when they popped into my head. It was difficult to become accustomed to relinquishing negative thoughts about myself and my life at the time, but I made the decision to follow through so I could get off the rollercoaster I was on and move forward as a happy, mentally healthy woman.

As each day passed, I consciously replaced my destructive thoughts with good ones more and more. I could feel a contrast happening in my self-esteem. I began relating to others in a different way and my overall disposition was improving. The further I dove into the material, the more energized I was, and in turn, good things were happening.

Prior to setting out on this journey, I was convinced that I naturally vibrated at a lower frequency. I believed it would take more work to rewire my brain. The ironic thing is that because I thought I naturally vibrated lower, I did! I was manifesting my own depressed state without any knowledge of doing so. When I came to that realization it was a game changer! Or, in my case, a life changer.

That moment was a turning point in my journey and life. I became aware of using the term 'cancel' to undo negative thoughts. Instead, I replaced it with a self-affirming phrase like, 'I am whole, strong, powerful, harmonious, and happy!'

I was shifting the paradigm of my menopause journey by changing my mindset. It was exciting! The work I was doing was retraining my brain. I was already doing it! I was already living it! I went through a menopause mindshift using my thoughts and mindset to improve my symptoms.

*My heart is open
to receiving all good
in my life now*

CHAPTER NINE

Finding Self-Love

The more I understood the universal laws and manifestation, the more I could really see how much I desired to be loved by others. I had never thought about loving myself. It just never occurred to me that I should love myself first and foremost. I never pieced together that my ability to love others started with loving myself first.

Even the work I have done in previous years with the law of attraction focuses on gratitude. I am so very grateful for my . . . whatever. I don't think I ever said that I loved myself. Sure, I was grateful for my life, along with this, that, and the other thing, but never grateful for the love I had for myself.

WOW! That was a huge revelation. How does one love oneself? Is it innate? Is it taught when we are young?

I always understood the outside forces that influenced how I viewed myself. How I was treated by my family, friends, and colleagues was always a factor in how I viewed on the outside, in physical terms. But I didn't realize how those outside forces affected the way I thought and felt about myself.

I mean, I get that the teasing I experienced as a child affected my self-confidence at times made me feel bad about myself, but I didn't understand the difference between those feelings and having love for myself.

I can see now how they have always been intertwined. Outside contributors made me feel bad about myself, which made me not like myself, and not liking myself led to lack of love for myself.

'I'm not good enough.'

'No one likes me.

'I must have something wrong with me.'

'I'm a weirdo.'

Maybe I didn't hear 'I love you' enough growing up. Instilling self-confidence wasn't on the parent checklist in my family. I don't think it was something that anyone in my family thought of when I was a child. I'm sure there are many children who grew up hearing the words 'I love you,' but mine wasn't a household that threw it around a lot.

I didn't grow up playing organized sports or being part of a Girl Scout troop. Summers were spent swimming, and I did more solitary activities than group ones. Friends were few, so I spent quite a bit of time with my elderly neighbours in my early teens. I visited with them and walked their dogs for them. We kept each other from being alone.

As a child, I was also a victim of molestation by a family member. I can't remember exactly, but I would guess it was about the age of seven. Victims often say they feel different from other kids, and I was no different. At first, I didn't understand the correlation between feelings of self-love and childhood trauma, but after going through it, I can see where the connection is. Something was stolen from me, and I was never getting it back. It has been something that is just there. It's a part of me, and maybe even part of who I am. At this point of my life, I choose to believe that it gives me strength. We survive many things during this life, and this was just one of those things.

Times really changed from my childhood to when I had my children. It was all about making sure they felt nurtured, had self-confidence, and knew they were loved. We read stories every night before bed, making sure the last thing we said was 'I love you,' and told them 'Great job' when they accomplished something.

They played soccer and hockey. They took dance and horseback riding. They were raised knowing how to be part of a team and get along with others. They had sleepovers and birthday parties. We made sure they felt safe.

It was also a time when having smart children was the 'in thing.' Every child was in competition with their classmates to have the best grades. It was a battle of the uber-smart when my kids were growing up.

I know my parents did the best they could, and I appreciate and love them for that. When I grew up, it was a different time to raise children. We were bathed, fed, and put to bed. We weren't played with and didn't have one-on-one time with Mom or Dad. Dad certainly didn't change, feed, or bathe us. He didn't make dinner, do laundry, or any other household chore. He was the breadwinner. Dinner was ready shortly after he arrived home from work, and he didn't eat Kraft dinner and fish sticks or homemade macaroni and cheese. We had those meals when he was on afternoon shifts.

If we misbehaved, we heard, 'Wait 'til your father gets home' from Mom, or 'Don't make me get up' from Dad.

We got the belt if we didn't listen, and the fear of God was instilled in us. As a side note, I threw away the belt when I was around eleven years old. The last time I got it was the last time I got it. I thought, That's enough of that, and threw it in the garbage. To my surprise, it never resurfaced after that.

Fast-forward forty-five years to a time when I don't recognize myself in the mirror and my mind starts reverting to that girl who didn't feel worthy. Suddenly, feelings I thought I had dealt with long ago were back and I didn't know how to process them.

I associated my physical appearance with love of myself. That included my weight, skin, hair, and overall body. I was convinced people would like me more if I looked good. Reverse that thought, as well. I believed I needed to look good so people would like me. Either way, I was using outside impressions of myself and seeking love outside of myself instead of inside me. I want to be healthy and well for me and no one else. Presently, not just on my journey.

I've heard manifestation mentors encourage the use of mirror work to improve self-confidence and self-love, but it wasn't something I had done a lot of. I couldn't look at myself in the mirror without finding a list of things that I didn't like about my body.

They say it is one of the best ways to begin to love yourself more, so I started trying it. 'Okay,' I thought. 'Is this really going to work?' I stood in front of the mirror naked and forced myself to look past what I didn't like in my reflection. Instead, I chose to say all the beautiful things about myself I could see.

I find it so interesting how the psyche works. At first, I saw just a couple of things like my eye colour and my nice ears. The more I did it though, the more my list increased to include so much more, including my calves, waistline, clean skin, cute feet, long legs, and so on. Something began to happen as I said these things to myself each day. It felt good. I felt good. I could feel my vibrational frequency rise as I repeated these beautiful words to myself about myself.

I was becoming more appreciative not only of myself, but those closest to me. I wrote down as many things as I could think of about everyone in my life. The more I wrote, the better I felt about everything. My attitude was changing. I was ascending, and it was a big step for me! It was healing for me because I could sense a shift in my reality, and I liked how I felt.

Doing mirror work alone has not miraculously healed me from years of self-doubt. I was on a beautiful journey of growth. I was going through another mindshift, and I was really learning what love was. I was embracing having an open heart, when I had been closed off for so long. Inner peace and calm came to be part of my daily life, where sadness used to reside.

What does this have to do with menopause symptoms? Everything!

I had hit rock bottom. How I felt about myself affected every aspect of my being. The worse I felt inside, the more terrible it was. I was in a vicious circle of feeling down, which only exasperated my hot flashes, sleeplessness, and lack of energy. The life was being sucked out of me with each passing day, and who knew when there would be an end.

Once I recognized and acknowledged that, there was only one way to go, and it was up! Learning to love myself has been the final piece to the puzzle of 'me.' I have visualized, meditated, written, and mirrored myself together piece by piece over the last year.

I have told myself that I am a Queen and I deserve to live my best life as much as anyone else. I feel her. I act like her. She was in me the whole time; I just had to release and unleash her.

I am a Queen
and I shine
brightly through
my menopause years

CHAPTER TEN
Tying It All Together

My big epiphany on my journey of self-discovery was that it's all connected! Our thoughts, feelings, emotions, views of ourselves, and how we view others are all intertwined in our being. We hold all these things within our bodies in one way or another and it must come out somehow.

Stress, for example, can affect the mind, body, and soul in such a profound way. Being under constant stress for a long period of time has been proven to cause pain, depression, physical ailments, even cancer. Yet, we do the same job, live the same lifestyle, and stay in the same relationships instead of thinking and focusing on what we really want out of life.

When women enter menopause, their bodies are stressed, and things go awry. Focus shifts to being outward to try to deal with all the changes going on, when really, it's all about what's happening inward. Our view of ourselves from the outside is skewed. We see ourselves differently. We think of ourselves differently. Who is she?

What if we go within instead? What if we work on what's happening inside our heads? After all, the brain is the control centre of our bodies. What if we can shift the way we think? What happens?

Incorporating lifestyle tools such as meditation techniques, frequency music, and practicing gratitude has reminded me of the power of the mind. When given the proper stimulation, the mind can do wonderful, miraculous things for us. It has certainly done miraculous things for me!

There is a quote from Bob Proctor that states, 'We have the ability to learn, unlearn, and relearn,' and I believe that this is an important phrase to remember.

I think about it in terms of perception. What we perceive is what we believe. Just because you were raised a certain way, lived in a specific house, and are part of a particular family, doesn't mean that you can't have your own style, your own personality, your own independence, and your own individual thoughts.

There is one thing at the root of every practice, and that is LOVE. Love makes the world go 'round' is the most powerful truth there is on the planet. We are born out of love. We are born into love. We are raised with love. We grow to love. We accept love. We die being loved.

The most important love is the love you have for yourself. Your inner voice may tell you otherwise, especially during menopause, when you don't recognize the person you see in the mirror. She can't be you. Who would love her? It's all about how you perceive her.

It's then that is the most imperative time to love yourself and show yourself-love.

Practicing meditation, music, and gratitude are only aids to bring you back to love. When you are in tune with love and are vibrating high, your thoughts do the rest. Your thoughts can tell your body to heal itself. They can instruct your body to function normally. Your thoughts can bring you wealth and the life of your dreams, including relief from your menopausal symptoms. Perception is everything.

You might think it takes a lot of time to meditate and write a gratitude list, but it doesn't have to. You don't have to meditate for hours. Some only meditate for five to ten minutes at a time. If morning doesn't suit you, then try at night. Daily is best, but if you can't practice daily, then just do it as often as you can.

You can also write out a list of things you are grateful for in as little as five minutes if you so choose. It's all up to you! Some people begin with writing down three things they are grateful for and may find they can add more to the list over time. Others dedicate an hour each day to meditation and gratitude. It's all in you. Who was it that said, 'If you really want to do something, you will find the time?' In this case, if you really want to change your situation, you'll find the time to help yourself. Helping yourself is really what it all boils down to.

I shared the various tools I used because I experimented with each of them separately and now combine the various techniques that have worked for me. I start with meditation and then listen to solfeggio music or Lucky Girl Syndrome affirmations while I write my gratitude list. I spend forty-five minutes to an hour altogether each day, because that's the time I want to dedicate to myself each morning.

Be consciously aware of your thoughts. Picture your body in its perfect state. Visualize yourself as you want to be. Affirm that you are healthy and well. Live your life as you see yourself in your thoughts and your body will comply.

I repeatedly tell myself I am healthy, well, and in perfect balance. I picture myself sleeping soundly, eating well, and exercising, and my body complies, reinforcing that the mind is a powerful tool.

Focused practice has relieved me of most of my symptoms I was experiencing. Continually visualizing myself in a healthy state, enjoying my life, and telling my body that my hormones are functioning perfectly has actually had a real effect on my symptoms. My immune system is healthy and well, and so on. I am well. I am well. I am well.

All of this reinforces the love I have for myself. It is the recipe to my success. I affirm that I am fantastic and amazing. I repeat affirmations to myself such as: my menopause journey is easy, and I love this phase of my life.

I embarked on this journey to share what I have experienced, because most of the literature and material I have seen on this topic focuses on which supplements to take, what medication works best, which exercises to do and foods to eat to reduce symptoms.

Rarely do I see someone encouraging other women to take the time to love themselves. Few speak of using your mindset to focus on improving your symptoms.

I'm here to tell you that if I can do this, so can you! There are hard days when you feel like you've been run over with a Mack truck and it's hard to just get out of bed. There are even days when it feels like the universe isn't listening because things aren't happening for you. I've had those days.

Those are the days I need to stop and check my vibration. Is it low? In essence, (in my opinion) during menopause, we get caught up in the symptoms and forget about life. Some days it's difficult to see beyond tomorrow.

The down days, the depression, the feeling shameful about the weight you've gained, repeated infections, changes in body chemistry, and the list of symptoms goes on and on. When you think about those things, it lowers your vibration, causing the universe to comply.

I discovered that even though I was writing down all the things I was grateful for, I didn't always believe them, and my vibration was low. I had to retrain my brain to focus on the good things about myself, my life, other people, and who I wanted to be. I wasn't the person I wanted to be.

I used the tools I had learned a long time ago in a new way to get me there. I allowed myself to slow down, take time out, relax, and calm my mind. It was in this calmness of mind that I was truly able to envision and start rebuilding my life.

It took some time, but gradually, I was able to regain my focus and think about things differently. I remembered that I was in charge of my own thoughts. I was healing myself from the inside out.

I saw myself as I wanted to be, which was healthy, powerful, and happy. I pictured myself in my favourite bikini lying on white sandy beaches. I was in perfect health.

I had power. I have power. I was powerful. I am powerful! I was strong. I am strong. I was healthy. I am healthy!

Those are the things I wrote about. These are the things I write about. Those are the things I remind myself of. This is the way I behave. This is how I think of myself.

This is what I want for you! This is what I want for all menopausal women.

Don't get stuck. Don't lose faith. Don't just settle.

Do keep going. Do have faith in yourself, God, the universe or whomever you trust. Do live your best life, using your thoughts to do it!

My hormones
are perfectly
balanced and in
complete harmony
at all times

Universal Laws

*T*concept of Universal Laws is rooted in metaphysical beliefs. These laws govern the universe and our interaction with it. Understanding these laws can provide insights into how to navigate life more harmoniously.

1. The Law of Divine Oneness

This law suggests that everything in the universe is interconnected. Our thoughts, actions, and beliefs affect not only us but also the people and the world around us. Understanding this oneness can foster compassion and empathy.

2. The Law of Vibration

According to this law, everything in the universe, including our thoughts and feelings, operates at a certain frequency or vibration. By aligning our personal vibrations with what we wish to attract, we can bring positive changes into our lives.

3. The Law of Correspondence

This law reflects the notion that patterns repeat throughout the universe, and our reality is a mirror of what's happening inside us. It suggests that by changing our internal state, we can change our external reality.

4. The Law of Attraction

Perhaps the most well-known, this law states that like attracts like. Our thoughts, feelings, and beliefs attract experiences and situations that match them. Focusing on positive thoughts can, therefore, attract positive outcomes.

5. The Law of Inspired Action

This law complements the law of attraction by emphasizing the need to act on your goals. While it's important to visualize and think positively, taking concrete steps is necessary to manifest your desires.

6. The Law of Perpetual Transmutation of Energy

This law suggests that energy is always in motion and can be transformed from one form to another. It implies that with the right energy and focus, we can change our circumstances.

7. The Law of Cause and Effect

Also known as the law of karma, it states that every action has a corresponding reaction. Our actions, thoughts, and feelings have consequences, shaping our future experiences.

8. The Law of Compensation

This law is related to the law of attraction and the law of cause and effect, suggesting that we receive what we give. It covers not only financial compensation but also the intangible returns of kindness, love, and energy.

9. The Law of Relativity

This law teaches that each person will receive a series of problems for the purpose of strengthening the light within. Our experiences are relative to others, and challenges are meant to be viewed as opportunities for growth.

10. The Law of Polarity

Everything has an opposite, and opposites are identical in nature but different in degree. Understanding this law helps navigate through the ups and downs of life by finding balance and integration.

11. The Law of Rhythm

This law states that everything moves in cycles and has a natural rhythm. Recognizing and aligning with these rhythms, whether they are in our personal lives or in nature, can enhance our experiences and understandings of the world.

12. The Law of Gender

This law suggests that masculine and feminine energies are present in all things and are necessary for creation and regeneration. Balancing these energies within ourselves and in our relationships can foster harmony and creation.

Bonus Law: The Law of Assumption

Created by Neville Goddard, the law of assumption is based on the theory of quantum physics, that everything in the universe is energy. The law of assumption states that by believing something already exists, you will manifest it.

WRITE YOUR OWN AFFIRMATIONS:

WRITE 10 THINGS YOU ARE GRATEFUL FOR NOW:

Resources

Website: "The 9 Solfeggio Frequencies and Their Benefits." MindEasy, October 27, 2023. https://mindeasy.com/the-9-solfeggio-frequencies-and-their-benefits/.

Assaraf, John, and Murray Smith. *The Answer: Grow any business, achieve financial freedom, and live an extraordinary life.* New York, NY: Atria Books, 2008.

Bisson, Shantelle. *Loving yourself without losing your cool a guide to help you get back to loving yourself unapologetically.* La Vergne, TN: YGTMedia Co. Publishing, 2022.

Byrne, Rhonda. *The Magic. London,* England: Simon & Schuster, 2012.

Byrne, Rhonda. *The Secret.* New York, London: Atria Books; Beyond Words, 2018.

Byrne, Rhonda. *The Secret to Love, Health, and Money: A masterclass.* New York, NY: Atria Paperback, an imprint of Simon & Schuster, Inc, 2022.

Cameron, Kathleen. *Becoming the One.* Mount Albert, Ontario: Hasmak Publishing International, 2021.

Canfield, Jack. *Life lessons for mastering the Law of Attraction: 7 Essential Ingredients to living a prosperous life.* Deerfield Beach, FL: Health Communications, 2008.

Gunter, Jen. *The Menopause Manifesto: Own your health with facts and feminism.* New York, NY: Citadel Press/Kensington Publishing Corp, 2021.

Richo, David. *How to Be an Adult in Relationships: The five keys to mindful loving.* Boston, MA: Shambhala, 2022.

Richo, David. *Triggers: How we can stop reacting and start healing.* Boulder, CO: Shambala, 2019.

Schwarz, Joyce A. *The Vision Board: The secret to an extraordinary life.* New York, NY: Collins Design : Distributed by HarperCollins Publishers, 2008.

Silva, José, and Philip Miele. *The Silva Mind Control Method.* New York, NY: Pocket Books, a division of Simon & Schuster, Inc. 1977.

I have shifted
how I think of
menopause, and
I feel great

About the Author

LISA R. TRIGGS is a trendsetter and the visionary behind *The Menopause Mindshift*, a movement dedicated to empowering women to take control of their lives during menopause. After enduring years of struggle, Lisa transformed her own experience with menopause by mastering her thoughts and now seeks to share her journey with others.

Lisa's mission is to help women manage and alleviate menopause symptoms through thought tools such as meditation, music, and gratitude. With a deep understanding of alternative methods, she emphasizes the importance of letting go of what no longer serves us to lead a healthier, more vibrant life during menopause.

Her passion for sharing her unique menopausal journey is driven by a desire to inspire other women to explore and adopt alternative methods to reduce their symptoms. Lisa excels in encouraging women to live their best possible lives, providing relatable stories and advice drawn from her own experiences.

Dedicated to spreading health and wellness during menopause, Lisa leverages her personal success with a positive mindset to help as many women as she can. She is determined to show that while the journey may have setbacks, the results are worth the effort.

Known for her compassion, kindness, love of travel, and dedication to her family, Lisa R. Triggs is a beacon of hope and support for women navigating the challenges of menopause. Through her efforts, she aims to give the gift of health and wellness, empowering women to take control of their lives and thrive during this transformative stage.